50 THINGS TO KNOW
BOOK SERIES
REVIEWS FROM READERS

I recently downloaded a couple of books from this series to read over the weekend thinking I would read just one or two. However, I so loved the books that I read all the six books I had downloaded in one go and ended up downloading a few more today. Written by different authors, the books offer practical advice on how you can perform or achieve certain goals in life, which in this case is how to have a better life.

The information is simple to digest and learn from, and is incredibly useful. There are also resources listed at the end of the book that you can use to get more information.

50 Things To Know To Have A Better Life: Self-Improvement Made Easy!

Author Dannii Cohen

This book is very helpful and provides simple tips on how to improve your everyday life. I found it to be useful in improving my overall attitude.

50 Things to Know For Your Mindfulness & Meditation Journey
Author Nina Edmondso

Quick read with 50 short and easy tips for what to think about before starting to homeschool.

50 Things to Know About Getting Started with Homeschool by Author Amanda Walton

I really enjoyed the voice of the narrator, she speaks in a soothing tone. The book is a really great reminder of things we might have known we could do during stressful times, but forgot over the years.

Author Harmony Hawaii

There is so much waste in our society today. Everyone should be forced to read this book. I know I am passing it on to my family.

50 Things to Know to Downsize Your Life: How To Downsize, Organize, And Get Back to Basics

Author Lisa Rusczyk Ed. D.

Great book to get you motivated and understand why you may be losing motivation. Great for that person who wants to start getting healthy, or just for you when you need motivation while having an established workout routine.

50 Things To Know To Stick With A Workout: Motivational Tips To Start The New You Today

Author Sarah Hughes

50 THINGS TO KNOW ABOUT TEACHING YOGA

A Practical Guide to Transform Lives

Ann M. Jayne

Cover designed by: Ivana Stamenkovic
Cover Image: https://pixabay.com/photos/yoga-adult-asia-exercise-girl-1822476/

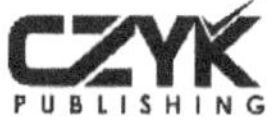

CZYK Publishing Since 2011.

50 Things to Know

Lock Haven, PA

ISBN: 9798578981241

50 THINGS TO KNOW ABOUT TEACHING YOGA

BOOK DESCRIPTION

Have you ever wanted to take a yoga class, but were afraid to because you can't bend like a pretzel? Would you like to learn how to relax? Would you try yoga if you knew that you only need to do what you can do?   If you answered yes to any of these questions, then this book is for you.

Most books on yoga tell you so much about its history, filling pages with information that, while interesting to some people, might be something that you have zero interest in. Or they get so technical and bogged down with words and jargon that you get glazy-eyed, confused, simply close the book, and place it on the shelf. Although there's nothing wrong with that information, it might not be what you are looking for right now, if ever. You just want to know how to practice yoga.

50 Things to Know About Teaching Yoga by Ann M. Jayne offers approaches and answers to these questions and many others that you might have to make yoga accessible and doable for absolutely anyone. Based on knowledge gleaned from yoga teacher training, workshops, videos, books and articles written by professional yoga teachers, physical therapists and other health professionals who practice yoga, Ann has presented ways to make yoga doable for you. She has placed her personal spin on it as a yoga teacher who cannot do all of the poses, but wants to help as many people as possible feel better physically, spiritually, and emotionally.

In these pages you'll discover that yoga is indeed personal. It is your practice. You customize it to how you are feeling on any given day. This book will help you learn that there are many ways to practice yoga and that you decide when enough is enough, when you have reached a limit, or when you can reach a little farther.

By the time you finish this book, you will know that you, too, can practice yoga. Any time. Anywhere.

TABLE OF CONTENTS

DEDICATION

I would like to dedicate this book to my mentor, Jennifer Henry, who first planted the seed about me becoming a yoga teacher. She gave me the best advice: teach what you know. I would also like to dedicate it to the faithful yogis who have attended my classes (14 years and counting), given me encouragement, and told me how much better they feel after my classes. You will never know how good that makes me feel.

ABOUT THE AUTHOR

Ann M. Jayne never dreamed that she would be a yoga teacher. After being dragged to a yoga class when she was 40 (with the perception that all yoga consisted of was chanting and chiming on a metal bowl), Ann continued to practice yoga, getting better and stronger, and leading a class after the instructor quit abruptly. She persevered, eventually teaching that particular class. Knowing there was much to learn, Ann began taking workshops, got certified, and became a professional yoga teacher in 2006. In 2010, Ann began her 200-hour registered yoga teacher certification courses and graduated in 2011. After 14 years of teaching, Ann, now an Experienced 200 Hour Registered Yoga Teacher (E-RYT200), is still learning; finding safer ways to teach her yogis so they can feel better and prevent or help injuries.

Teaching yoga classes allowed a flexible work schedule for Ann while she raised her two sons, Ian and Justin. When she is not teaching yoga classes, Ann enjoys writing, photography, riding her horse, hanging out with her dogs, rescuing dogs and helping the Animal Rescue League of Okemah, and trying to be the best wife, mother, sister, friend and Christian that she can be. She lives in Edmond, Oklahoma with her husband David, beagle (Ajax), rescued Treeing Walker Coonhound (Bowie), and horse (Harry).

She is currently on YouTube as Ann Jayne Doable Yoga, Facebook and MeWe as Ann Underwood Jayne (check out "Doable Yoga" in her Facebook Albums), Parler @Amjayne, and LinkedIn.

INTRODUCTION

*"If I'm losing balance in a pose,
I stretch higher and God reaches
down to steady me. It works every
time, and not just in yoga."*

Terri Guillemets

P

erhaps you think that yoga is silly, that all people
do during a yoga class is say chants that no one can
understand while sitting cross-legged on a mat. That
was pretty much what I thought yoga was for a very
long time. When I got married to my husband David
in 1986, I began taking aerobic dance classes at the
Edmond YMCA. Yoga classes were offered after the
aerobics classes, but I never stayed. It's just chanting,
remember?

Fast forward to 2002. I was 40 years old and the
mother of two boys, ages six and two. I had been
taking kickboxing classes at a local gym. I loved it,
but my shoulders started rebelling from the constant

punching. So Susan, my horse trainer and friend, told me to come to a yoga class she had been taking. I reluctantly agreed, not knowing what to expect.

When we started class, I recognized the teacher as the one from the YMCA years ago. Susan whispered to me, "We call her the yoga Nazi." What? Nazi isn't good! Nazi is never good! But class started and Hana, in her Czechoslovakian accent, began teaching yoga. It was a tough class but I stuck with it. I came back, too. And just as I was starting to not dread it and kinda sorta get the hang of it, Hana left and went to another gym.

The new teacher, Jennifer, taught differently, teaching an Ashtanga-based type class. (FYI, there are about as many flavors of yoga as there are churches.) I was 40. Nothing hurt and the fast-pace of the class and the dozens of chaturangas (yoga push-ups) was undaunting. I really enjoyed Jennifer's classes and we became good friends.

There was another yoga class at the same gym with a different teacher and I attended it, too. It was very different but also very good. The teacher left abruptly, like, right-before-class-was-about-to-start abruptly. Several of the women in the class, who also went to Jennifer's class volunteered me to teach.

Why me? Why not you? Or you over there?
Everyone but me took a step backward.

So I taught the class by basically copying
Jennifer's class. Then I began subbing for Jennifer
when she needed me. As I advanced and learned
more, Jennifer told me something that I was not
expecting. She told me that I should be a yoga
teacher. I argued that I didn't know as much as she
did, I couldn't do as much as she could, I still needed
a wall for handstands and headstands, I couldn't sit in
Lotus Pose because my hips were so tight.

Jennifer simply told me to teach what I know. She
told me not to worry about teaching the poses I don't
know how to do. She said it's like teaching the Bible
to someone. You don't start with Revelation. You
just tell them about Jesus!

Well. I waited a while because another teacher,
Shay, had been hired for the other class and I really
liked her.   She also asked me to sub her classes.
When Shay left a couple of years later, I became the
teacher for her class. She also got me hired at a
YMCA in Oklahoma City to teach her yoga class.
This led to another yoga class at another YMCA! I
enrolled in a weekend workshop to get a certification
through YogaFit, and then I was teaching 4-5
classes/week!

Was I nervous? Sure I was. I didn't want to copy Jennifer's class, so I attended some workshops and bought one of the instructor's books that broke down the poses (with great photographs), showed modifications, told what muscles and parts of the body were working, and gave contraindications (health issues that might prevent someone from doing this pose or causing more pain/injury). I was discovering that most people wanted to open their hips (me, me, me!), had sore shoulders, tight hamstrings, or low back issues. So I scoured and studied and highlighted the book. Then I began typing up yoga practices that dealt with a particular issue. For example, I collected the poses that help the low back and put them in an order that flowed from one to another. And the rest, as they say, is history. My "cheat sheets" are still saved on my computer!

I incorporated some of Jennifer's class into mine but developed my own style. When people asked me what type of yoga I taught, I told them "non-denominational" or the "Ann Jayne" style of yoga. After 14 years, my classes keep evolving. I'm 58 now and my shoulders will last through about 3 chaturangas. Most people in my classes don't want to do the crazy stuff; they just want to stretch or help their shoulders, hips, knees, back, or all of the above.

I've given up on structuring a class in advance because when I do, invariably someone will ask if we can work on something that doesn't have much to do with what I planned. So I just make it up as I go along and recycle it through the week.

Along my journey, I decided that I want to include everyone and make my classes "doable." I don't care if you are eight or 80, are the perfect weight or you exceed the perfect weight. No one is excluded. That, dear readers, is yoga.

1. WHAT IS YOGA?

The word "yoga" means "to yoke" (to link or connect) the breath, body and mind. This can occur during movement in a pose or sitting quietly.

Some teachers chant. Some start and end a class with "Om," which sounds like "Mom." I do not chant or even say Om in my classes. I do not know any of the chants so I'm not going to chant something that I cannot say or know what it means.

Yoga is not a religion. Yes, it has Hindu roots. It also has YMCA roots from 150 years ago. I have been to some workshops and read some books/articles and the instructors have trained in India and appear to make yoga their religion. I am not one of them. I think that you can make anything your religion. To me, yoga is a very important, calming, and at times, invigorating, form of exercise. It manages to exercise the mind as well as the body. It is also something you can practice off the mat, meaning in your everyday life. We will get to that later.

2. ASANAS

Most yoga poses have Sanskrit and English names. Every Sanskrit name ends in "asana," which means "pose." Asana is pronounced "ahs-uh-nuh" or "ahs-uh-nah." It could depend on what part of the country you are in, taking drawls and dialects into account. So, for example, Child's Pose is called Balasana ("buh-los-an-uh or "ball-os-an-uh"). The beginning of the Sanskrit name usually corresponds to what the pose looks like or what that thing is called, such as an eagle (Garudasana) or camel (Ustrasana). However, you really have to use your imagination for Gomukhasana, or Cow Face Pose.

Some yoga teachers will only use the Sanskrit names. They may use the phrase "moving through our asanas," meaning the yoga practice or class.

I use both names. For certain poses, it is much easier to use the English name. Downward-Facing Dog (Down Dog for short) is easier to say than Ahdo Mukha Svanasana. Likewise, Pigeon Pose is much, much easier to say than Eka Pada Rajakapotasana. I once had a yogi in my class ask me why I didn't use the Sanskrit name for Pigeon. So I did. I'm sure I jumbled it up, but she got the idea and agreed that "pigeon" was much easier. Other poses have similar-sounding names, like Chair Pose (Utkatasana) or Standing Forward Bend (Uttanasana), so English names may be better for the class. Usually I will tell people to get into Chair Pose and then say "Utkatasana" as a friendly reminder. For one particular pose, Savasana, I mostly use the Sanskrit name because it means "Corpse Pose." I think that is creepy so if I don't say Savasana, I call it Relaxation.

3. LISTEN TO YOUR DOCTOR BECAUSE I AM NOT A DOCTOR

If you have underlying health issues, please consult your physician before you begin practicing yoga. More than likely, he/she will tell you that it is fine. However, there may be certain poses that you should not do. For example, if you have glaucoma, forward bends and any poses with your head lower than your heart should be avoided or severely modified.

Many people have come up to me before or after class and told me about a medical issue they have. They also ask me what they should do. I tell them to discuss it with their doctor. If it is something like "simple" knee pain (not bone on bone or torn ACLs) and bending their knees hurts, I will advise them to not bend their knees much, maybe not at all.

4. SAFETY FIRST

Going hand in hand with a doctor's advice is my teaching philosophy that safety comes first. Always.

I always give modifications to a pose. I always inform the yogis in my class (give them "permission") that they can modify or even omit a pose for any reason. I will not yell at them or kick them out of class. No one gets called out. I will compliment someone on their pose, but I will also compliment the whole class as well so that, while Betty is rocking a pose, Fred won't think his pose looks like crap if I don't say anything to him. Everyone's pose is what it is.

Some things are obvious. If someone comes in wearing a boot, they probably shouldn't do balance poses on that leg. Common sense. That is the number one safety lesson. If you know you shouldn't, or physically cannot, do a pose, do not do it. It really is that simple. If someone is too scared to try or do a pose, that's fine. Maybe they will try it later. Maybe they will try a little bit of it. Maybe not. It is okay.

5. NO INTIMIDATION BECAUSE NO ONE IS PERFECT

Aside from safety first and using common sense, be sure you check your ego (large or small) at the door. Maybe someone is running low on self-esteem. Maybe someone is not athletic. None of that matters. Sometimes big, inflated egos will get a dose of reality because they think "yoga is easy."

Probably the hardest thing about yoga is not comparing yourself to others. As a teacher with the tightest hips in the world, this is a tough one for me sometimes. I won the "Tight Hips Award" in a yoga workshop once and was privileged to sit on not one, not two, but three blankets to help open my hips. So looking out into the classroom and seeing someone sit in Lotus Pose (Padmasana), sitting cross-legged with their feet tucked in on their opposite hips, makes me a little jealous. I will tell the rest of the class if they need to see what open hips look like, that I'm not the poster child. Without singling someone out for criticism, I'll comment how beautiful their open hips are and I'll tell them that I'm jealous in a good-natured way. I did this to a girl once. She practiced beautiful poses and when we sat down cross-legged, her hips opened and her knees were on the floor. I told her I wished I had hips like hers. I'm pretty sure that made her feel better because I got a big smile in return.

Face up to the facts that someone will always be more flexible than you are. Someone will be thinner. Someone will be younger. Face up to these facts and drop them like a bad habit. There are gymnasts and ballerinas in yoga classes. They will pretty much be able to do anything. Okie dokie. Good for them. If you aren't auditioning for Cirque du Soleil, what does it matter? You are in yoga to feel better, physically, mentally, and spiritually.

When we are working on something challenging, say, like splits, I remind my class that there is not anyone from *Yoga Journal* outside, waiting to take a photo of someone doing the perfect splits. Believe me, they have their own people for that. Maybe your yoga neighbor's legs look like one long line and his sit bones are on the floor. Again, good for him. Admire it and focus on your splits.

I have had NFL football players in my classes. They were a hoot. For people you might think would have an ego in spades, they didn't. They were friendly and kind and helpful. They were serious about practicing yoga, too. One day I wore a tee shirt to class that had their NFL team logo on it. They thought that was pretty cool.

There have also been people in my classes who felt the need to tell me that my classes weren't challenging enough, that I needed to do this or that, or that they didn't get anything out of it. Okay. Thanks. I have had someone tell me that I shouldn't have let a really heavy person in my class! I told her that they absolutely need to be in my class!

A man who used to come to one of my classes told me that another instructor told him that yoga was not for him (he had knee issues) and that he should just leave! I told him that I would never tell anyone to leave, short of them threatening me with bodily harm or setting the room on fire. He kept coming back. His knees got a little better.

I do not care what color someone is or what religion they practice (if any). I do not care what someone's tax bracket is or what zip code they live in. I do not care how many marriages they have had or to whom they are attracted. I do not care if they look like a supermodel or like a sack of potatoes. I do not care how old they are.

My job is to teach. It is not to judge. It is not to criticize. It is not to suck up to someone. In my classes, everyone is equal. Period.

6. YOGA ATTIRE

While this isn't really something I teach, I wish Susan had told me before my first class not to wear a baggy tee shirt and sweat pants. While the sweat pants themselves weren't really an issue, the tee shirt kept falling down around my head when we would practice forward bends or down dogs. It was really a pain. I ended up tucking it in, and then purchased some yoga pants and tops.

So as a general bit of advice, clothing should be stretchy and form-fitting if possible. It doesn't have to be skin tight, but you don't want to spend half of your time pulling your shirt back down. Sweat pants can get hot, too, especially if it is a very active class.

You don't have to spend a fortune on yoga clothes, either. Discount stores and athletic/sporting goods stores carry exercise/yoga clothes. That is where I shop. I refuse to spend $80.00 for a pair of yoga pants when I can find some that work just as well for $20.00.

Yoga is generally practiced barefoot. I have never noticed my feet, lack of toenail polish, or chipped-up toenail polish as much in my life as I have in my yoga classes. It is possible to practice in tennis shoes, but remember that you are on a mat and it can get scratched up or torn more easily from shoes or gravel in the shoes. If you are in the park and decide to do a few standing poses, it's fine to have on your shoes. You probably don't have your mat with you anyway, so just breathe and practice and enjoy your poses.

There are yoga socks with the toes separated. This is really good for your feet. So they might be something that you would like to try.

7. BYOM

Along the lines of safety first, I highly recommend that you purchase your own yoga mat. Most gyms provide yoga mats. However, they are used multiple times a day, by multiple people. So bear in mind that these people are sitting on the mat. They are standing on the mat. They have their hands on the mat. They sneeze on the mat. They cough on the mat. They drip sweat on the mat. They fart on the mat.

Yoga mats can be purchased at discount stores or athletic stores for a reasonable, and sometimes cheap price. I am not a germaphobe, but a yoga mat is like a 6-foot petri dish. Chances are high that it isn't cleaned after every use. It's rolled up and tossed in the closet with the other much-used petri dish mats.

Spend about $15.00 and get your own mat. You can clean it as you need to and you know that you are the only one who has been on it.

Additionally, to practice proper yoga etiquette, try to avoid walking or stepping on someone else's mat. It is included in their personal space.

8. JUST BREATHE

With the housekeeping, personal hygiene, and safety issues more or less out of the way, the key takeaway from yoga, in my opinion, is the breath. As I told you, yoga links breath with movement and the mind. I tell people who are new to yoga, "If you don't get anything else out of the class, just breathe."

We have all probably heard the great advice, "Breathe and count to 10." That is kind of yoga in a nutshell.

In yoga, we breathe through the nose. That keeps the warm air inside and it can go to the muscles. It can help you focus, too. The goal is to make the inhales and exhales the same length. New yogis may inhale to the count of three and exhale to the count of three. Veteran yogis might be able to count to six or eight or more.

Unless we are working on specific breathing exercises, most of the time we don't hold our breath. Oh, people might actually hold their breath, not meaning to. That is why I remind everyone to breathe. We do hold our poses and breathe while we are in these poses. Most of the time in my classes we hold the pose for five or six breaths. Sometimes we hold them for 10 breaths. I will remind new yogis that they may be taking eight to ten breaths if their breaths are shorter than "seasoned" yogis.

When all else fails, or when frustration or exhaustion sets in, or when the outside world creeps in, just breathe.

9. YOUR BONY REALITY

Bony reality refers to how the skeletal system is built. My bony reality is that my hips are tight, tight, tight. The heads (the ball) of my femurs, with very little neck, are crammed into the hip sockets with very little wiggle room. I have the X-rays to prove it. Lotus Pose for me is basically impossible. There is really nothing I can do about it. I can, however, bend over and touch my palms to the floor or squat down with my heels on the floor because there isn't a long neck between my femurs and the heads of my femurs, where it connects to the pelvis. Give and take.

My left hip is now made out of titanium, and soon my right one will match it, thanks to genetics compounded with arthritis. But that "only" relieved the pain. The artificial hip had to match my old, worn-out, arthritic hip. Muscles extend and flex according to the bone structure.   My left hip actually will open a bit more, and the great thing is that it does so without immense, throbbing pain. Can I get my left foot on my right hip for Half-Lotus? No.

Another example of bony reality is that short spinae processes make a deep, full, backbend hard to do, if not impossible. So, there really isn't anything to do about that either except accept it.

So…now what? Refer to #10, #11, and #12. It isn't the end of the world if I will never do a Lotus Pose.

10. DO WHAT YOU CAN DO

So many things tie together in yoga: safety, breathing, modifying a pose, omitting a pose, checking the ego at the door, not comparing yourself to anyone else. My teaching philosophy is "Do what you can do."

Face it. There are some of us who will physically never be able to do certain yoga poses. There is nothing wrong with that. If Steve weighs 400 pounds and has no desire to lose weight, he is not going to be doing any handstands or headstands. That's reality.

However, he can do some poses standing or sitting. He can breathe. Some yoga poses are very doable for Steve.

Perhaps Alice is bedridden. She isn't paralyzed, but is too weak to walk. Alice can lay in her bed and work her arms and legs, open her hips, point and flex her feet. Alice can breathe.

Basically, anyone who comes to any of my classes can do some yoga poses. Their pose may not look like a textbook Warrior 2, but it may be the best that they can do.

11. MODIFY, MODIFY, MODIFY

I teach my classes so that they are doable for anyone. One thing that I stress in every class is modifying a pose. Modifying a pose means tweaking it a little to meet your physical needs. That can include using props (see #12). Whether or not you are using a prop, you might need to adjust one side a little. Or a lot.

Let's say that Camille can't touch her toes in a Seated Forward Bend (Paschimottanasana) due to tight hips (forward bends help stretch the hips), low back pain, or tight hamstrings. All Camille needs to do is bend her knees. A little or a lot. That will relieve the pressure wherever it is. I teach my yogis to always have at least a tiny bend in their knees. It can help prevent injuries later on.

One of the biggest problems I see with Standing Forward Bend (Uttanasana), is that people, mostly men, bend straight over, loading their weight on their low back. They usually can reach their knees, maybe their shins, because they have tight hamstrings. I watched a young basketball player do this one day while I was substitute teaching at a high school. I told him to bend his knees! Please! He did and was able to reach a little farther.

Chaturangas (yoga push-ups where the elbows bend backwards to work the triceps), short for Chaturanga Dandasana, which is also called a Plank, require much upper body strength and core. They can also be murder on the shoulders if they are done improperly or if you do a zillion of them. To modify, put your knees on the floor and do a Half-Plank, then lower your upper body to the floor. Your shoulders will thank you.

12. USE PROPS

Doing what you can do most assuredly implies using yoga props. We have yoga blocks and straps. You can also use a wall or chair. Sometimes an extra rolled-up yoga mat helps. I tell my classes that God made props for a reason. Use them!

Blocks are great for forward bends or standing poses like Triangle (Utthita Trikonasana, Trikonasana for short). If you can't reach your toes, you might be able to reach a block. For sure you should be able to reach your thighs. That is also an option since your thighs are a prop that are always with you. The block can be placed on any level. Once you have progressed with the block at the tallest height, lower it and give yourself a challenge, making the distance to the block a little greater. For Seated Forward Bend, if your head won't reach your shins, put a block or three on your shins. Build a little tower if you have to.

Yoga straps help you stretch a little deeper. They are great for putting around your foot so you can lift your leg a little higher, whether you are sitting or standing. You can stretch the strap out between your hands and lengthen your side stretch or buckle the strap around your upper arms and use it for resistance in a Down Dog. Maybe you aren't able to clasp your hands behind your back or go into a full bind. A strap helps that. Straps are a good way to open up your chest and heart and get a little deeper into a backbend, too.

Chairs or walls are useful with balance poses and perhaps other standing poses. Having a wall within reach of your fingertips or hand can be a big confidence builder and help you psychologically. They are a safe way to practice headstands and handstands. Most of the people in my classes know that when we are working on balance poses, I will invite them to use the wall. The "veterans" usually head on over to the wall without the invitation.

Walls are very beneficial for standing poses such as Triangle (Trikonasana), Warrior 2 (Virabhadrasana II), various forward bends and Half-Moon (Ardha Chandrasana). Even if someone normally doesn't have trouble with these poses, the wall gives you the feeling you should have in the middle of the room: it doesn't move and you aren't able to "cheat." It can be a really great workout and most people really enjoy it when I tell them to take their mat and all of their goodies to the wall.

A chair can serve the same purpose as a wall. Standing next to or behind a chair gives you the reassurance that you are close to it in case you need to put your fingers or hand on it. Chairs, and even the wall, are good to do Half-Dogs in case you should not, or cannot, bend over in a regular Down Dog.

Rolled up yoga mats or blankets are great to sit on to help tight hips. You can tell if your hips are tight by sitting cross-legged. If your knees are higher than your hips, congratulations. Welcome to the Tight Hip Club, of which I am president. Elevating your hips by sitting on a bolster of some sort helps even things out. Remember, I got to sit on three blankets at a workshop! So if you need some help, you need some help.

13. STRUCTURING A YOGA CLASS

As I mentioned in the introduction, I used to plan all of my classes. For shoulders, we will do this, this, and this pose in a particular order. Same for hips, low back, legs, etc. I would teach the class and over time I became very familiar with which poses helped what issue/ailment/body part the best.

So I would plan my classes, writing them down and going over them in my mind on my way to work. (Today we are really going to work on our hips! It will be great!) And then I would get to class and someone would ask if we could work on our hamstrings or shoulders or low back. Or all of the above. Now I had to think on the fly; everything I had planned (and I am not a planner or list maker) would go out the window. I had to check the recesses of my mind and remember what poses were going to help what particular body part, or parts, someone needed help with on that day.

Basically I stopped planning my classes. As I learned more and more, through workshops, videos, and articles and my yoga books, I'd gather that information together for my classes.

I know some teachers who teach the same class all of the time. Ashtanga classes are the same but they are in a series of six (Primary, Intermediate and Advanced). I've only done the Primary Series. It is enough! Bikram yoga classes (practiced in 105° rooms) are the same as well (26 poses practiced twice). Maybe you like doing the same thing. It is familiar. You learn it. That's good.

However, I don't teach that way. Along with knowing which poses help for which issues, I structure my yoga classes in a way that starts off slowly, letting people warm-up and stretch. Then the class can get "busier" with deep stretching in standing poses and balances, allowing people to get warmer and stretch more. After that it is time to go to the floor for some seated poses and more deep stretching before slowing down and preparing for Relaxation (Savasana). I do that with my classes, ensuring that there is a nice, fluid flow and segue from one pose to the next.

I usually recycle my classes at different gyms. I may tweak it here and there so it is a little different, or because I forgot something and had to come up with another pose. In the end, all of my classes are different. They are never exactly the same. I've had people ask me if we could do the class we did three weeks ago! We surely could if I remembered what we did!

While my classes flow, they also vary. For instance, I teach classes sometimes where we never stand up. We stay on the floor the entire time. Other classes we might work one side for 15-20 minutes and then work the other side. If I have an end goal, a particular pose, we will spend much of the time getting our bodies ready for that pose.

Sometimes I throw in "party trick" poses. If it is right before a holiday, I tell my class that they can impress their family and friends. There are always some laughs, sometimes some groans, and always the option of sitting and watching. As I tell my yogis, "I don't want you to get bored."

14. GETTING INTO AND OUT OF A POSE

Since we practice safety first, I teach different ways to get into and out of poses. I inform the class that they will probably be different on each side. Your left side may be tighter or looser than the right side or your balance may normally be better on your right side than your left side. Joan may float right down into a Triangle Pose on her left side. But when she has to go into Triangle Pose on her right side, she might need to make some adjustments and arrive from a different route, perhaps bending her knee as she goes down, then straightening it as she opens into Triangle Pose.

Coming out of a pose is the same. It may vary for each side and for what is going on with a particular person that day. I think it is more important to come out of a pose safely and carefully. If the pose is difficult or one that someone is not particularly fond of, they may be in a hurry to get out of it. Hurrying out of a pose might cause someone to cut corners and end up hurting their back or hamstrings or something else.

Take your time. As I frequently tell my yogis, "It's not a race."

15. PREPPING FOR A POSE

Some poses need preparation. The groundwork needs to be laid, caution needs to be taken, bricks need to be added.

When I am teaching a class with an end goal, we work on other poses that will help us get into that pose. If we are headed to a Headstand (Sirasana), we will do extensive core work. For Splits (Hanumanasana), we work on hips and hamstrings until it is time to split. If we are working on a full bind in Extended Side-Angle (Utthita Parsvokanasana), we may do the pose two or three times on each side, delving deeper, doing what we can do, until perhaps some of us can bind our hands behind us, maybe with the use of a strap or grabbing our shirt. Many times I will tell the class that I have a method for the madness that we are doing. It might be met with some quiet mumblings (which I'm not privy to) followed by suppressed snickers or a loudly whispered, "Oh. Great…"

I have to know how to teach these specific poses, so I will work on them at home. A good one is Crow Pose (Bakasana). It is a forearm balance, relying on upper arm and core strength. As I'm teaching it, I demonstrate it using a block, for my perch. I also tell everyone, because it can be a little scary balancing on your forearms and not wanting to faceplant, that I worked on it at home with a bunch of pillows around me! We build up our arm and core strength before attempting it. We go through it step by step by step, with the invitation to stop at any step. It is very satisfying to watch someone lift both feet off the block or floor for the first time, perhaps if only for a second. Then everyone is rewarded with some seated stretches, a twist or two, and Savasana.

Take your time. Practice. Breathe. Then fly!

16. VISUAL AND VERBAL CUES

When I am teaching, I have my mat at the head of the classroom. I face the class so I can look out and see if someone needs help. I think it is friendlier, too, so the class isn't staring at my backside the whole time. I prefer to give direct and helpful verbal cues. Very rarely will I make a physical adjustment on someone. I have my reasons.

The first one is one I learned when I began teaching. I can't remember what pose we were working on, but someone in the class wasn't quite getting it, so I stepped off my mat and walked over to help them. On cue, everyone in the room left their mat and followed me! Hmmm. All eyes are literally on me! Now if there is a need for me to leave my mat and go help someone, I tell everyone to "stay put."

One of the very first workshops I ever attended was an Ashtanga workshop. I thought I was a badass since I had been going to Jennifer's classes. However, after no less than 80 Chaturangas, I learned that I wasn't really a yoga badass. When we finally got to a seated pose, the instructor "adjusted" me. We were either working on a Seated Spinal Twist (Sage) Pose or "Screaming" Pigeon Pose. I don't know how you say "screaming" in Sanskrit but my guess is that Indians with tight shoulders or quads scream as well as Americans with tight shoulders or quads.

In Sage Twist (there are several versions to this seated twist), you are on your sit bones, one leg is bent with the foot on the floor and the other leg is extended. If the right leg is bent, you twist to the left. You can wrap your right arm around your right shin and bring it behind the knee. The left arm reaches around the back and maybe you can clasp hands, or maybe not. In Screaming Pigeon, let's say that the right leg is bent and the left leg is extended behind you. Bend the left knee and sit upright. The left hand will grab the left foot and perhaps wrap around it. The right arm will reach over the head and anyone with rubber shoulders can reach back and clasp the left hand. Looks good on paper. Or in *Yoga Journal*.

Whichever one we were in; I wasn't quite able to clasp my hands. I was sort of close. The teacher came over, grabbed both of my arms, pulled (jerked) and got my hands to clasp. Yeah. I wasn't quite ready for that. I didn't blurt out any obscenities, but they were rumbling up my throat and headed towards my tongue. Although nothing snapped in two, no blood spurted out, and I didn't fall over in an unconscious state, I just wasn't ready to go that far. The instructor should have known that. Here's another point to consider: men are usually stronger than women. He was bigger than I was and also did about 6,000 Chaturangas each day. As I said, he should have known better.

It is okay to gently help someone if they ask, stopping when they say it is far enough. It is quite another thing to physically grab a person and pull, or wrench, her deeper into a pose she may be, or oftentimes may not be, ready to deepen. Ouch. Or worse…lawsuit.

One other instance occurred when I was teaching Half-Moon Pose. It is one of my favorite poses, at the wall or away from the wall. A woman in my class was in the pose but wanted to open her hip more so she asked me to help. She was standing on her right leg and the left leg was lifted, with the left hip opening. I stood behind her, placed my left hand on her left hip and my right hand on her extended left arm for support. Then I gently eased her left hip open.

"OW!"

I thought of some quick swear words as I let go. "I'm sorry!" I said.

"Oh, it's okay. I just hurt my hip earlier. It wasn't you."

Sigh. Okay. I didn't know she had hurt her hip, but I pretty much made a vow right then and there that I would not physically adjust people ever, ever again.

Besides the risk of injury of getting someone deeper into a pose, another reason I do not physically adjust people in my class is that some people just do not want to be touched. Period. Their mat is their personal space and territory. I respect that. That is also one more reason I don't partner people up in class like one instructor used to do. Besides the "NO TOUCHY!" aversions, if I don't know everyone in the class, I probably won't want to pair up with them and let them invade my space.

The instructor who had us pair up did it to work on standing poses such as Triangle. So we would be mirror opposites, back-to-back. If we had worked up a sweat, well, our sweat was intermingling. Gross. Our butts were pressing against each other. No thanks.

I have also been to workshops where the instructor, a "famous" yoga teacher at the time (who was later exposed for sexual abuse and harassment), had us partner up and our personal space was thrown out the window. We were in Butterfly Pose (Baddha Konasana), seated with the soles of our feet together. Or thereabouts. It is a hip opener. People with open hips have their knees go to the floor. Mine were about 10 feet above the floor (this wasn't the workshop where I won the Tight Hip Award).

The instructor told us to have our partner reach under and grab the flesh around our sit bones, yes, in there, and pull the flesh back so the hips open more. Oh it worked. (To this day, I'm good friends with my partner. Not because of the intimate moments we shared, though.) But really? I'm sorry, but I'm not teaching my class to play grab-ass and I'm pretty sure they would say no, report me, and I would be fired. So if we are working on this, I tell my yogis to move their own flesh away from their sit bones.

Now you have my reasons for being "hands off." I take what I learn and verbalize it, telling the class what muscles we are working and giving analogies, sometimes interjecting humor into it. For instance, if we are really stretching our arms, I'll tell them to imagine there is a great big diamond right there and they can get it if they just reach a little bit farther. Or if we are reaching forward with both arms, say, in Chair Pose, I'll tell them to hold their hands like they are holding a bowl of Snickers. Incentive, whether it is diamonds or Snickers. It paid off, too, as one yogi did indeed bring me a bag of Snickers!

If someone is a visual person, like I am, I tell them they can look at me and see what I'm doing. Some of the yoga rooms where I teach have mirrors in them and I think they are a great tool so you can see what your pose looks like and any adjustments that you make.

I have had many people tell me how much they appreciate my cues and descriptions. I really appreciate that because I do not want to sound like a broken record all of the time. I have found that, sometimes, repeated cues are like reading a Bible verse that you have read 100 times before. At just the right moment, it clicks. You get it. A whole new world has just been opened.

17. ASK QUESTIONS

Asking me questions during a yoga class is not taboo or forbidden. I want people to ask me questions if they aren't getting it or if they want to know if their hand placement is okay, etc. That is how we learn. I tell them to ask me questions.

One really good example is usually when we are squatting. Squats are based upon one's bony reality in their hips and/or ankles. I usually go through my Squat Sermon about your hips deciding how far down you'll go, if your heels are on the floor, or if your feet turn out (and make sure that your knees turn out, too). Sometimes I don't say everything.

Now, one thing about my hips. Besides being extremely tight, they are constructed so that my heels touch the ground in a squat.

"Are my heels supposed to be on the floor?" is a common question I'm asked. Not all of the time. But I'm guessing that the person who asks it is visual and they see my heels down. If I haven't given them the Squat Sermon, now is the time to do so.

Once I tell them "No, your heels don't have to go down," they are usually satisfied. In fact, it's usually a good time for me to have the yogis who do have their heels down to lift them up and get a good foot stretch and balance a bit.

I may not have every answer, but I'll try and answer the questions as best as I can.

18. CHILD'S POSE

Perhaps one of the most important poses is Child's Pose (Balasana). Whenever I am teaching beginners, I make sure we do Child's Pose at the start of the class. I let them know that Child's Pose is a very important pose. It is restorative. It is calming. It may be a "go-to" pose in that a yogi can go to Child's Pose at any time during the class in lieu of another pose. Child's Pose is also an alternative to Down Dog as well as a segue to safely push back into Down Dog.

There are also modifications to this pose. I enjoy having my knees apart, giving some room for my ribs between my thighs. Arms can be extended towards the top of the mat for a really good stretch, or the forearms can be on the floor. For a big shoulder release and upper back stretch, bring the hands around by the feet. Ahhhh!

Even yogi veterans enjoy Child's Pose. I try to incorporate it at least once in my classes, for a bit of a rest. However sometimes I forget and I get reminded. Once I was teaching a somewhat aggressive class and after we did some extensive movement and stretching, I called out for everyone to go to Child's Pose.

"Finally!" someone mumbled.

"I thought you forgot all about Child's Pose," someone else grumbled.

Point taken.

19. HEAD, SHOULDERS, KNEES, AND TOES (AND NECK)

In yoga, we work everything. Maybe we get to all, or most, of it in one hour. Maybe we just work on one thing, or a couple of things that tie in together. Each pose usually works other things besides the specific body part we target.

Shoulder pain and/or tightness is a common complaint. Stress is stored in our shoulders. At any given time during the day, stop and inventory your shoulders. Chances are, they are pulled up by your ears and are tight. Simply let them go. Release them to where they should normally be. I remind my yogis of this all of the time. Sometimes we sit and breathe, letting our shoulders go where they go. Or I will remind them in a pose to release their shoulders, especially if we are reaching up with our arms. Bend the elbows. Modify.

Knee pain is another culprit. When we are doing some serious knee bends, or maybe we are on our hands and knees, I inform people to pay attention to, and listen to, their knees. Sometimes I'll simply call out for "knee people" (there are also "shoulder people," "hip people," and "low back people") to modify, to know their limits and when it is okay to bend a little deeper. But I caution everyone as a group by telling them that if they have bad knees, new knees, need new knees, or want to try and avoid new knees, to use caution or even avoid a pose.

I also address neck issues in my classes. We hold our heads different ways and that affects our neck. Pulling the chin in, sticking the chin out, or lifting the chin can tighten the neck muscles. Check yourself out right now. I learned a very helpful way to ease stiffness and pain in the neck at a Doug Keller workshop. If you hold your neck in one of the ways I just mentioned, put your fist under your neck. Rest your chin on your fist. Congratulations! You just put your neck in a neutral position! You always have your fist with you, so whenever you feel your neck tensing up, see how you are holding your head. I remind everyone of this in class. Except I tell them to imagine holding a caramel apple (with nuts) under their chin.

During poses such as Triangle, I give everyone the option to look down at their front foot, look in the direction they are opening up to, or up at the ceiling. See which one your neck likes better today. Tomorrow may be different. Some poses such as Shoulder Stand (Sarvangasana) and especially Plow (Halasana) may need to be avoided entirely if there are neck injuries. Avoid putting undue pressure and stress on your neck. Keep that caramel apple with nuts with you at all times.

20. HIP HIP HOORAY

I have mentioned my poor old hips enough. Besides shoulders, hips are the other place where we shove our stress and anxiety. They are like suitcases and we keep shoving crap in there. Do another inventory and see what is going on with your hips. There is a good possibility that you are clenching them and you don't realize it. Stretching and opening hips is the most popular request I get. I'm always up for opening hips.

If the hips are tensed up, simply release them. Stop crossing your legs, too. That tightens the hip flexors. Cross your ankles instead. Breathe. If you have to sit for long periods of time, get up and move around!

I often tell my class to exhale into their hips, especially when we are laying on our backs. We also massage our hips, getting into the hip creases where the thigh meets the pelvis. In some standing poses, such as Triangle or Parsvokanasana (easier to say than Extended Side Angle Pose), I may tell everyone to put their hand on the hip of the leg that is stretching back, providing a hip opener, and tell them to press down towards their foot.

Hip openers can be a blessing or a curse. They can be quite painful for some people to practice, even though they will probably feel better after working on hip openers. Even if you don't have tight hips, as we get older, things just don't stay as stretched as they should. Some things don't work quite the way they used to. That's the aging process. Maybe your hips don't stretch or open like they used to, if they ever did. Stretch and open them, anyway.

21. FIND THE TIME TO MOVE

Movement is vital. More so as we age, but it's important to kids, too. It is imperative to stretch, bend, and open at least once per day. Even if you only have 10 minutes, utilize that 10 minutes.

Some yoga studios are sticklers about being on your mat when class starts. I understand that. It can disrupt the whole class when someone comes strolling in, looking for a place to land. Even though I teach at fitness centers and not private studios, I would prefer it if people can get there on time. I do understand that things, such as traffic or trains or the dog getting loose can cause someone to be late.

I have never told anyone to not come in because we have already started. Usually, they apologize at the end of the class. Sometimes they tell me that it is a real struggle for them and they consider not coming to yoga. I always affirm to them that they are welcome and 10 minutes is better than nothing. I'm rewarded with them telling me that they do indeed feel better after coming to my class. There are some people in my class who have told me that they will always be a few minutes late because of their schedule, or that they have to leave early. I'm glad when they tell me so I know what to expect. I tell them I'll leave a spot for them! I also appreciate it when they tell me they have to leave early, as I want to make sure they aren't hurt or offended or intimidated.

During my classes, I will tell often tell the whole class that 30 minutes, or 10 minutes, or five minutes of yoga is better than no yoga. I'll even give them tips for poses they can do a few minutes a day or while they are going about their day (See #23), keeping yoga very, very doable. Then I tell them that if they hold a pose, such as Chair Pose, for one minute (about 10-12 breaths) and they do this 10 times during the day, they will have practiced yoga for 10 minutes!

If you have to be late for whatever reason, use proper yoga etiquette and enter the yoga room quietly out of respect for the teacher who is yammering away, and for the other yogis. I used to teach a class at a gym and there was a man who attended who was always late. When he came in, everyone braced themselves because after slamming the door, he unfurled his yoga mat like a stagecoach driver cracking a whip. SNAP! Once he got his nest made, he left again, slamming the door. He would come back in about 20 minutes later, I assumed, because we had a good chunk of the standing poses out of the way. Don't be this guy. Please.

22. WE AREN'T JUST STANDING AROUND

Mountain Pose is a standing pose. The Sanskrit name is Tadasana. Think "Ta Da!"

If someone walked by and saw us in Mountain Pose, they might think that yoga is a piece of cake because all we are doing is standing around. That is partially true, but we are working a great deal while we "just stand around."

Tadasana, like Balasana (Child's Pose), is a pose that you can use to re-group, re-focus, or take a breather. Sometimes while I'm teaching, we will stand in Mountain Pose for several breaths. For giggles, and a balance check, I have everyone shut their eyes. Just the simple act of closing one's eyes puts a whole new spin on things. You might feel yourself wobble or sway a little bit.

This pose is also a great time for my "Bucket Sermon." I have several sermons I preach to people intermittently. During my Bucket Sermon, I tell everyone to imagine that their pelvic girdle, say from your belly button to your pelvis, is a bucket full of water. If you stand with your hips pushed forward, water will slosh out the back. If you stand with your butt sticking out, water will slosh out the front. If you stand with your right knee bent, water will slosh out of that side and vice versa. Standing correctly in Tadasana keeps the water in the bucket.

Another way I teach Mountain Pose, for a change of pace, is to have everyone stick a block between their thighs and then imagine that they are pushing it out behind them. This gets the thighs to roll inward without letting the knees push back and hyperextend (ouch!). The calves are pushing forward, the feet are planted, and the ribs are lifting up while the head reaches toward the ceiling.

Now do all of that without a block. Like I said, there's a lot going on in Mountain Pose. Ta Da!

23. PORTABLE POSES

I guess most poses could be done anywhere, although you might get some stares if you dropped down to Pigeon in the middle of the grocery store. However, there are some poses that you can do throughout your day and no one will really know that you are practicing yoga. What if they do? No worries!

Mountain Pose is one of those poses. You can do it anywhere that requires standing. It isn't as tiring as shifting from one leg to another, especially for mothers who are carrying a baby in an infant seat on one hip, a large diaper bag with everything but the kitchen sink in it on the opposite shoulder, while holding the hand of a toddler. I tell my yogis it is perfect when you have to stand in line or when you are standing up singing in church.

Tree Pose (Vrkasana) is a balance pose, and I inform my yogis that it can easily be done while you are standing at your counter cooking (but not when you are brushing your teeth) or washing dishes, or even when you have a free minute and maybe some wall space. A seated version can be done while you are watching television or riding as a passenger in a car.

Something that usually elicits laughter is when we squat and I tell the class this is perfect to do at the grocery store. Just pretend you are looking for something on the bottom shelf! It is great for stretching the hips and low back, and I have even done it standing in line at the store.

Other poses, such as Warrior 3 or Half-Moon can be incorporated into picking something up off the floor, cleaning horse stalls (check out my YouTube video on Portable Poses), or vacuuming (I prefer cleaning horse stalls).

If you have a minute or two and some wall space, you can do a Half-Dog and a Plank. Throw in some triceps pushups (mini Chaturangas) and knock out 10-12 of them. I tell my class this is great to do when you walk in a room and forget why you walked into the room!

Some of the poses can also be done right before you go to sleep or when you wake up. Bring one leg into Tree Pose for a hip opener to start or end your day. Place your feet on the mattress and tilt your hips up and down, working the spine in a small Cat/Cow, which is really good for your back. Twist your knees to one side and then the other. Relaxation (Savasana) is a great way to calm down and drift off to sleep.

24. THE FLOPPERS

I think one of the best articles I ever read (I think it was in *Yoga Journal* years ago but I'm not for certain) related to flexible and inflexible people. This goes along with comparing yourself to others in the yoga room.

In this article, the author called the flexible people "floppers." He stated that they are naturally flexible and can simply "flop" into a pose without any effort at all. The others aren't floppers at all. Nothing about them flops. They have to work and work at a pose.

This is where it gets really good. While the author appreciated the floppers, he had compassion for and enjoyed the "nonfloppers" because they really had to work at stretching even half an inch further. When they were able to see improvement, opening, and flexibility, they were ecstatic.

I enjoy telling this to my class from time to time, for reassurance and to boost their confidence and the ego that they left at the door. I need it for affirmation for myself, too. When I tell them this, it is nice to see them smile, get some hope, and stretch a little farther.

Cheers to the nonfloppers!

25. TAKE CARE OF YOUR FEET

In the equestrian world, there is a saying, "No hoof, no horse." If your horse has bad hooves, his mobility is limited, there can be immense pain, and perhaps even no options to keep living. The four hooves are holding up several hundred pounds (ponies) to a ton or more (draft horses). The hooves are vital.

Our feet hold us up, too. They carry us around, sometimes while they are crammed into high heels that look pretty but that's about it.

Yoga can be really good for your feet. Practicing without shoes lets you utilize your whole foot.

I will teach yoga classes devoted to our feet. We massage them. We curl our toes under and sit on our heels. We roll up our yoga mats and step back and forth on the mat with one foot, causing it to spread out and use most of the foot. We roll our feet on balls to help the plantar fascia. We wiggle our toes. We spread our toes apart. Even if it is not a class devoted to our feet, I will remind everyone to make sure that they aren't gripping with their toes in standing poses (especially balance poses) and to wiggle their toes while we are practicing seated poses.

The hips and knees are connected to the feet. Sometimes knee or hip pain can be associated with the feet. So I make sure, usually at least once in every class, that we notice that our feet, knees, and hips move together.

Extend your right leg. Turn the toes to the right. Notice that your right knee moves to the right and that your right hip opens a little bit to the right, too. This is important!

The knee should track towards the little toe. If your knee goes the other way, it won't end well for your knee. This is emphasized in certain poses. Safety first, remember?

In Warrior 2 (Virabhadrasana II), step back with your right leg and turn the right heel to the left. The heels should be lined up as if they are on a straight line. The left knee will be bent a little or more, maybe bending over the ankle but not going past the ankle. This depends upon your knees, so modify. Your torso will be facing the right, arms are extended out from the shoulders. I make sure, pretty much every time I teach Warrior 2, that the front knee, in this case, the left knee, tracks toward the little toe. This is especially crucial as we open up. The right hip will open. Some. If it opens too much, the left knee will rotate in to the right and not be going the same way as the foot. So I tell everyone to put their left hand inside the left knee and push very gently. We may not get a big hip opener, but we won't get a big knee injury, either!

The same goes with Triangle even though the front leg is straight (maybe a slight bend to the knee). The knee needs to track towards the little toe and not roll in.

For our old friend, the squat, if your feet turn out (whether the heels are up or down), make sure that the knees go the same way as the feet. You get an inner thigh stretch as a bonus.

When you are in Mountain Pose, make sure the knees aren't knocking together. And when you walk, let the knees follow the feet.

Take care of your feet. Get a pedicure or at least soak in the bathtub. Slather them with lotion and elevate them when you can. You want to keep your horse going as long as possible.

26. FIND YOUR BASE

Whether you take riding lessons, practice martial arts, do gymnastics, play tennis, whatever, most things require a set of fundamentals. Everything builds on the basics. They are the groundwork. To me, yoga is no exception.

For years, many yoga teachers taught that in a certain pose, say, Chair Pose (Utkatasana), the feet need to be together. Same with Mountain Pose. That's fine. Until you wobble. I began keeping my feet hip distance apart. I became more stable.

Look at a chair. The four legs aren't together. Look at a mountain. The base is the widest part. It makes sense, to me, then, that we need to practice with our feet at least hip distance apart. So I began incorporating that into my yoga classes. I've noticed that some of the teachers in the new yoga training videos I watch are doing this, too.

Sometimes I will teach a class where we flow from Mountain Pose to Chair, then step back to Warrior I and 2, then throw in Triangle and Extended Side Angle, stepping back to Down Dog. We will do this in a series of three, starting with feet together in Mountain Pose and Chair, then shorter stances in the standing poses. FYI, in Down Dog, you always want the feet at least hip-width apart. The next time the feet will be hip-width in Mountain Pose and Chair, and a longer and wider stance in the standing poses. The last time has the feet mat-width in all of the poses. It is then that I give the class their options to customize their poses, putting their feet where they need them and lengthening or shortening their standing poses where they need them.

Usually, older people need to have a shorter stance in the standing poses. They may not be able to stretch farther. They feel safer in a shorter stance. I will also teach classes where we shorten the stances. Believe me. It is not easier. You still have to work those legs and sometimes when they are closer together, you will definitely feel it. Taking a longer stance ends up being a treat!

27. COUNTERPOSES

Many poses necessitate a counter pose, or opposite movement. For example, after working on backbends, a forward bend can feel absolutely delicious. After many forward bends, a gentle backbend might be just what you need.

The big thing I teach regarding counterposes is taking care of the hands. If we are gripping blocks or straps, or using our hands for weight-bearing, as in Down Dog or Planks, Cat/Cow, or forearm balancing, we need to turn our hands in the opposite direction for a bit and stretch them.   This is a good way to ward off carpal tunnel issues, too.

I make it a point to tell everyone that if they hold their hands in the same position for a length of time, as in gardening, playing tennis, golfing, riding a bike or horse, or typing at the computer or playing video games, to take a few minutes and open up the hands (my Hand Sermon). Turn the palms to the ceiling, curl the wrists back and forth, stretch the fingers apart, gently pull down on each finger. Basically do the opposite position on your hands. Take a break.

28. TWISTS

Twists are a great way to work the core, stretch the upper torso, and give the internal organs a nice massage. They can help with circulation, too.

Many of the poses we practice have a twist. Triangle has a Revolved Triangle (Parivritta

Trikonasana) as well as others. Anything with "Parivrtta" means you will revolve, or twist, it.

Whenever we practice backbends, I always follow them with a twisting pose. Sometimes we follow after each backbend, other times we flow through the poses and then do a nice, long twist. If the practice is focusing on the core, twists are incorporated.

I have a sermon for twists, too. The most important thing to know is that twists do not involve the low back. Ever. Period. Right up there with this is that twists may not be for some people with back issues. Once again, consult your doctor.

When we are working on twists, usually seated twists, I have everyone face forward and put their hand, say the left hand, on their bellybutton. Then we draw in the belly button on an inhale, engaging the core. As we exhale, the upper back, chest and shoulders twist to the right. With the left hand on the belly button, yogis can know that they are not straining the low back. They are twisting what should twist. We do this on every inhale and exhale, perhaps twisting deeper as we exhale. I remind them that it can be hard to take a deep breath in a deep twist. The benefits of twists are wonderful!

29. FINDING BALANCE EVERYWHERE

The first thing to understand about balancing is that it isn't just standing on one leg. The seeming inability to stand on one foot does not mean that you are clumsy.

When you check your ego at the door, try to check everything that is going on in your life at the door as well. At least for an hour. Stress, anxiety, worrying about things, forgetting to do something, yelling at the kids, or a host of other things that happen in our lives affects our balance.

Of course, standing on one leg is a great deal of it. Wobbling around is fine. Everyone does. When you feel the most off-balance, unless there is an underlying medical condition, that is the perfect time to work on your balance.

Perhaps you are struggling to stay on one foot. So you have to set the lifted foot down. Big deal. Get back into the balance and carry on. It is hard to try and balance when we see our yoga buddies wobbling around, too, thanks to mirrors and our peripheral vision.

Often we will practice some of the standing balancing poses while laying or sitting down. Maybe balance isn't involved at all, or else you have to balance on your side, so the worst thing that happens is you roll onto your stomach or back. Practicing these before we stand up, and even after, can build confidence. Often we use a strap to help us, too, standing or laying down. Standing Extended Leg Stretch (Utthita Hasta Padangusthasana) is a great one to do laying down and get those hamstrings to stretch and hips to open. Do the pose standing up, perhaps using a strap or the wall, and you get all of the benefits, plus balance!

I remind my yogis when we are balancing that some days you have it (balance) and some days you don't. Yes, it is that simple. You might nail a perfect Dancer Pose (Natarajasana) during class and in an hour, or tomorrow, you can barely lift a leg off the floor, much less bring it behind you and hold it with your hand.

Sage advice regarding balance that I picked up in a workshop (I can't remember who said it) is, "If you fall, you're human. If you get back into the pose, you're a yogi." People like to hear that.

Focus. Engage your core. Use the wall. Get back up if you fall. Balance.

30. KNOW WHEN ENOUGH IS ENOUGH

Doing what you can do and modifying a pose go hand in hand with knowing when you have reached your limit. Perhaps it is physical and something, say your shoulder, is telling you this is it. Listen to your body. Perhaps it is mental and today you just aren't there or you don't have it together and it's not going to get together.

Stop.

Back off.

Omit this pose.

This might be a perfect time to crawl into Child's Pose and hang out a while.

You have a brain and indicators and warning signals from your body. Use them. Be safe. When you are ready, you can reach a little farther and stretch a little deeper. One day at a time. One pose at a time. Just like yoga isn't a race, it also isn't "Simon Says." Everything we do is optional.

Know when enough is enough. Know when enough is good enough.

31. POP GOES THE WHATEVER

When I tell people to listen to their bodies, I'm usually referring to listening to what their muscles or joints are telling them regarding pain, strain, that's far enough, don't do this, etc. However, listening to your body can be literal, too.

One day when I was teaching, I had everyone go into a squat. I couldn't have planned this or choreographed it if I had tried. As the whole class began to lower into their respective squats, a collective POP! POP! POP! erupted from nearly everyone's knees, including mine. Everyone laughed. It was a funny moment.

Hips pop. Elbows pop. Knees pop. So do backs and ankles and shoulders and necks.

Corn popping means you get a nice treat in a few minutes. Joints popping means that they are dry and need some synovial fluid. Think of the oil can for the Tin Man in *The Wizard of Oz*.

The best way to get the synovial fluid flowing, aside from being 5-years-old, is to keep doing what you are doing. If your ankle pops when you roll it around, keep rolling it around until the popping stops

or gets much quieter. The joints are getting
lubricated, without an oil can.

32. RESTORE AND RELAX

I used to teach a class after school at my sons'
school for the teachers, office staff, and
superintendent. We worked on standing and seated
poses. One day they came in and all of them had
obviously had a rather crappy day. So we got on our
backs and I began to help them get restored. Deep
stretches and breathing followed by Legs-Up-the-
Wall (Viparita Karani) actually turned into Legs-
Thrown-Over-the-Couch-Cushions, leading into our
final relaxation, Savasana. This was just what the
doctor, well, yoga teacher, ordered. That pretty much
became the norm for our classes, with the addition of
some Cat/Cow poses, as well as Half-Planks and
Down Dogs for strength and building bone density.

There are days when I still teach a totally
restorative class. Sometimes we never stand up;
everything is done on our backs, stomachs, or seated.
People tend to absolutely love it.

Most people truly enjoy Relaxation (Savasana),
too. However, for some, it can be the hardest pose to

do. What's so hard about laying on your back and relaxing? Well, for some men who used to be in my class, nothing. As soon as they hit their backs on the mat, they began to snore. That is relaxing!

For others, it can be excruciating. Relaxing in a room full of people might be the culprit. Being still might be a challenge. Stilling and quieting the mind is the biggie, though. Grocery lists, errands that need to be run, fixing supper, taking the kids to 40 different activities, something you said or had said to you might all be factors competing with, literally, your peace of mind.

Periodically, we begin class with Savasana. No one ever complains. I will also incorporate Savasana throughout a class, perhaps every 15 minutes with a short two-minute Savasana intermission, or after we have worked one side robustly and before we get to the other side. Again, no one complains. No one really wants to get back up, either!

During Savasana, I will lie down as well, mainly out of respect for the class. Personally, if I'm trying to relax and someone is walking around the room or sitting up, it might give me the creeps. Not to mention if they are talking, telling me how relaxed I should be. That actually happened in a workshop once. The teacher would not stop talking!

On occasion, as I'm about to bring people out of Savasana, I will sit up. I have noticed a few people who are laying there as stiff as pokers. Or they look like water simmering and about to boil. Savasana is clearly not their thing. At least not today.

It is so important, though. Turning your mind off is the hardest thing. Learning to do nothing for a few minutes doesn't jive with our twenty-first century lives. Just like balance, though, it is something that all of us absolutely need for at least a few minutes every day. Be still… God tells us to do that.

33. CHILD'S PLAY

As I've said, yoga benefits everyone. Several years ago, I taught a summer kid's yoga class. Herding cats doesn't even compare to this. Oh, I had taken a YogaFit Kids Yoga workshop. I learned some fun things to do, like games such as "Bowling For Butterflies" to play. What I didn't learn was that the kids will take over the class if allowed.

So after the first class, I had to form a new battle plan. I scoured thrift stores and toy stores for small toys, such as little chairs, army men, and animals. I put them in a bag and the next time we had class, I had the kids form a circle with their mats. They took turns pulling out an item that corresponded to a pose. So that's the pose we did. We had balancing contests. We played Bowling for Butterflies extensively. (I had a ball that I rolled to the kids, who were sitting in Butterfly Pose on their mats. They had to dodge the ball by raising their knees out of the way. Whoever got bumped by the ball was "It." They loved it.)

When the class was over for the summer, I had already made a vow that I would never teach a kid's class again. I subbed a few years later, though. It was equally as fun because I wasn't the regular teacher and didn't do the class exactly like the regular teacher did. For example, one little girl asked me if we were going to "Fairy Land" today. I asked her what that was and she explained it. I told her, "No." She sat down and pouted.

My biggest takeaway is that the most important thing to do in a kids yoga class is have the kids divided by ages. The 12-year-olds are more focused; the three-year-olds want to run around the room. It's like oil and water.

I do want to point out that yoga is great for kids. I'm sure they thought I was some old geezer and I couldn't bend like a pretzel like half of them could. No worries. We could still have fun.

Teaching yoga did come in handy when I was a substitute teacher. When I subbed for the elementary school, we took breaks and stood up and stretched, did some animal poses and tree poses, breathed, and "got the wiggles out." Well, most of the wiggles.

34. CHAIR YOGA

The other end of the spectrum is teaching senior citizens in chair yoga classes. I took a workshop about this and purchased books about it, too.

Modification is key here. We only hold poses for two or three breaths. Many of my senior yogis are 90 years old; however one is 96 and another one is 99! The 99-year-old tells me every time that her back hurts. She said if it keeps hurting she will stop. Fair enough. She also keeps her purse with her and will root through it during class. She is gone lickety-split when she sees the activities director go by with a cart of donuts. If I live to be 99, I'm eating donuts, too.

They are childlike, in a way, and I love teaching them. It is interesting hearing about their lives. One woman, who has now passed away, told me she grew up in Kentucky. Her family used to pack a lunch and sit outside Churchill Downs to see the movie stars who were going in to watch the Kentucky Derby. She said they were too poor to pay admission so they listened to it outside the gates and ate their lunch.

I used a playlist with songs from the 60s once. As I looked at everyone, I realized that most of them were 40 years old when these songs came out. I might need to make a Big Band playlist.

Chair yoga can be practiced seated or standing with the chair next to you or in front of you. For my octo-and nonagenarians, we stay seated. That doesn't mean we don't work. The first thing I want them to do is to just move. So I pare down the number of breaths we hold a pose or the time we lift our arms. Most of them are pretty good at keeping up. I also figured out how to do Chaturangas by having them put their hands on their thighs and push up and down four times. Sometimes we put our hands on the chair seat and lift our rears up and down an inch or two. We also do sit ups by leaning back into the chair and then lifting up. I'll combine the sit ups and pushups, too.

And on Bingo Day, I learned to wrap class up a little early so they can get set up for Bingo! I tell them what we worked on will help them reach better and maybe kick their neighbor's Bingo card away if the neighbor is winning. Not too Christian, but they

laugh and a couple nod their heads in approval
("That's a good idea!"). The stakes are high: $0.50
or cans of food, so I have to help them in any way I
can.

When I left one day, I heard someone grumble, "I
think Ann was trying to kill us today." Things that I
teach them may help build up a little strength and also
help them if they fall.   I'm not trying to kill them, but
rather to keep them moving and winning at Bingo.

35. PRACTICING YOGA FOR TWO

Yoga can be practiced during pregnancy.
However, I strongly encourage pregnant women to
make sure their doctor approves. Some women are
obviously pregnant when they come into class.
However, I'm not going to suggest that someone is
pregnant unless I see a baby's head crowning.
Usually they tell me, especially if they aren't too far
along. I will ask them if they have been practicing
yoga. If they have, they usually know what they can
do but I caution them against twists and aggressive
core work. And absolutely no inversions. For those
who have never done yoga before, I tell them the
same thing and to please check with their doctor.

I have watched some videos about yoga during pregnancy. Some of it is obvious, like not laying on the stomach when the woman is quite a ways into her pregnancy. Forward bends need to be modified with the legs farther apart so there is room for the baby. Open twists, facing away from the legs are okay. Twisted Triangle and others where you face the leg, however, are a no-no.

Common sense and safety should always prevail. I've never had to deliver a baby and I really have no desire to break that record.

36. ROCK AND ROLL AROUND

At the beginning and end of class, and intermittently during the class, I have everyone lay on their backs and pull their knees to their chest. It is basically a reverse Child Pose. I have them rock side to side over their sacrum. When I have them widen their knees, we rock back and forth over more of our backs, getting into the middle and upper back.

Pushing into Sphinx Pose, literally on our stomachs with our forearms on the floor, helps put the low back into a gentle back bend. Pushing the hips and elbows down makes it a little deeper. Then as a bonus, we rock back and forth on our hips. This can also be done with the arms crossed and the head resting on the arms.

One other good spinal roll out I teach is to pull the knees into the chest, extend the legs, and grab behind the knees. The core must be engaged and we rock back onto our shoulders and then up to our sit bones. Sometimes we do this several times and it is a good core buster and a good way to vertically roll out the spine.   I caution anyone to avoid this if they have back issues.

37. ENGAGE YOUR CORE

Our abdominal muscles, the deep core muscles, are crucial in yoga. Strong core muscles can support us as well as our low backs, helping to prevent injury. While some poses, like Boat Pose (Navasana) specifically target the core, the core is an active participant in all of the other poses as well. (However, in Savasana, we get to release and relax the core along with everything else!) Some poses, such as Headstand, very much depend upon a strong core and should not be practiced until the core is warmed up and strong. Twists are great for the core as well.

If you want one of the best core exercises in the world, do some Planks. Besides working the core significantly, Planks and Down Dogs work nearly every muscle in our bodies.

The core muscles we utilize are not the "6-pack" muscles.   They are much deeper than that.

The best way I have found to engage the deep core muscles is to gently draw the belly button toward the spine. This gets into those deep muscles. I remind everyone, without trying to sound like a broken record, in nearly every single pose, to pull their belly buttons to their spines. I might change it up for Tadasana and tell them to think about moving their hips towards each other.

I tell everyone that they can hold their core in whenever they think of it. It is a Portable Pose, too. All you have to do while standing, sitting, walking, watching tv, whatever, is to simply draw in your belly button to your spine. In fact, no one will probably know that you are doing it.   You will know and your low back will know. It will thank you.

38. YOU PROBABLY WON'T LIKE EVERY POSE

Boat Pose (Navasana) is a pose that combines balancing on the sit bones with deep core work. There are variations and modifications. Regardless, I really don't like it and I let the class know it. I have my favorite poses, such as Pigeon, Triangle, Half-Moon, and Wide-Legged Forward Bend (Prasarita Paddotanasana).

I'm sure if I went around the room, I'd find out who likes what and who doesn't like what. Sometimes it is evident, with "ugh," "yuck," "ahhh," or "yes!" It is okay to not fall in love with every pose. Some of them are really challenging, even with modifications. Other poses are more "fun" than the others. Many times, the poses we dislike are actually poses we need to practice. Maybe the poses are disliked because they are indeed, challenging.

In yoga, positivity is important. If there is a pose or five that some people do not like, it is actually okay. It does not mean that negativity abounds, but rather maybe fear of injury or a previous bad experience are the reasons. Modifications might help ease the sting or dislike, too. We can feel better afterwards. Perhaps, once the pose is practiced and a better outcome happens, it might not be met with consternation or fear again. Once the pose has been practiced, the yogi can feel accomplished. It is over and they survived.   In my classes, no one is ever forced to practice a pose they don't want to practice. They can simply find another pose to do, or watch us.

No one has to absolutely love everything about yoga. That is okay.

39. PRACTICE OUTSIDE

For a totally different perspective, practice yoga outside. Ditch the music and let the birds and breeze provide the soundscape. I have led a number of classes outside, on spacious front porches and in city parks. While the grass might not provide even footing and makes standing poses and balancing poses a little trickier, it does provide a soft cushion for poses on your hands and knees and seated poses.

If you go to the beach, practice yoga. Listen to the surf and breathe in the salty air. If you go to the mountains, practice yoga. Listen to the birds and breathe in the crisp, cool air. Your own backyard can be an oasis as well.

Outdoor yoga can fill your senses. You're breathing fresh air, not stuffy, recirculated, indoor air. You can focus your gaze, drishti (drish-tee), on something besides the same four walls. If it is warm, a gentle breeze is the perfect way to cool off.

For me, the best part of teaching and practicing yoga outdoors, wherever it is, is Savasana. You can take a quick nap as you listen to the birds or perhaps a squirrel. You can also stare up into the sky and watch the clouds. If you're under a tree, look at the branches and leaves from a totally different perspective. Watch as the wind blows the leaves and grass.

This is experiencing an ongoing miracle. The leaves turn colors, dying and dropping off to save water for the tree in the winter, then budding and blooming again in the spring. The clouds shift shapes and move across the sky. The ocean waves roll in and out. Mountain meadow flowers form a colorful canopy over your resting soul. Breathe it in!

40. PRACTICE WITH A PARTNER: HUMAN OR ANIMAL

Although I've told you that I don't teach classes where people partner up, it is good to practice with a partner. It doesn't have to be a hands-on experience. Your partner can be a helper if you are working on a particular pose, such as Headstand, and help you get up into it safely. Sometimes it is just nice to have someone to practice with.

Canine, feline, and equine (see #41) partners can "help," too. Sure they may get in the way, but they can still be a comfort and source of joy and companionship. My dogs, Bowie and Ajax, appear in a few of my Doable Yoga videos on YouTube. I have never practiced yoga with a cat as my husband is really, really allergic to them.

There's nothing quite like getting a nice, wet kiss from your canine companion to give you the warm fuzzies and lower your blood pressure a little. That probably doesn't happen in a yoga classroom.

41. GET BACK ON THAT HORSE

In #29, I told you about falling out of a pose and getting back in it. "Get back on that horse" is a phrase that means to keep trying. Rome wasn't built in a day, and for you, perhaps some of your poses aren't either. Don't give up.

You can also literally get back on that horse and practice equine yoga. If you are fortunate enough to own a horse, or have a friend who does, there are modifications of poses that you can do in and out of the saddle. Make sure the horse is well-broken. Unless you are a seasoned horseman or horsewoman, I do not recommend trying some of this on a green-broke two-year-old.

Give the horse a big hug. Practice a few poses standing next to the horse, avoiding sweeping and sudden arm movements. Horses can see nearly 360 degrees, which is why they usually see something behind them that we do not see. Use the horse for your Half Dog or Warrior 3, making sure the strength is in your arms and you are lifting away from the horse, leaving your hands lightly on your equine partner so you don't push him away.

Once you have warmed up a bit, you can try some poses sitting on the horse. Some poses can even be done at the walk. The horse may wonder what the heck is going on, especially if you are reaching for the opposite stirrup in a Triangle Pose. I pretty much guarantee you that the horse won't mind if you practice poses while he is standing. My horse Harry, who is an absolute diamond, doesn't mind at all. As Susan, my trainer friend who roped me into yoga, told me, "Standing is Harry's best event."

In Chair Pose, I teach to let the weight sink into your heels. This is an aspect of riding as well. So let your heels sink into the stirrups (like they should do anyway) and come into a Chair Pose, resting your hands on the crest of the horse's neck or his shoulders. Now you can get the true meaning of putting the weight in your heels. It will be more of a balance pose, too, so your core and quads are going to be put to work. Your calves will notice this, too.

Although I have never taught a yoga class specifically to riders, I have a friend who is working on getting an equine yoga class together at the stable where she rides.

Giddy up, yogis!

42. LET GO

Your yoga practice, whether you are practicing alone or in a group class, is a place to let go of whatever may be bothering you. Sure the problems will be there an hour later, but you have a respite for a bit.

Letting go, like checking your ego at the door, is hard. Whether you are experiencing something in your life or trouble/fear with a pose, try and let go. If you have a case of the "I Can'ts" (not an actual physical issue that is preventing you from a pose) and that is preventing you from getting deeper or farther into a pose, let go. Breathe. Practice by yourself. Ask for help in class. I have helped people when class is over many times. I do not mind at all.

Long before *Frozen* and "Let It Go!" came along (in my opinion the most annoying Disney movie and song that I have ever seen and heard), letting go seemed not to be an issue with me. But it all came together on particular weekend several years ago. I was taking a riding lesson on Harry and something was bothering me. It was affecting my riding. Horses are smart and intuitive. They pick up on things. Harry was picking up on whatever was going

on with me. Susan told me to pull up and breathe.
Yes, I was a yoga teacher and here was someone
telling me to breathe! She told me to let go of
whatever it was. Let. Go. She had me ride around
with my feet dangling out of the stirrups for a while.
When I put my feet back in the irons (stirrups) later, I
was able to accomplish whatever it was that I was
working on.

That same weekend, I had my yoga teacher
training classes. Guess what the theme was? If you
said, "Let go," you would be correct. Relax.
Breathe. Let go.

To compound things, our sermon at church was
about…letting go. Let God.

OKAY! I get it!

Is it hard? You bet it is.

Face it. There are things we cannot control at all.
Fortunately, I'm not a control freak so control of
everything isn't something I deal with on a daily
basis. But underlying fears or suppressing problems
or worrying is something I deal with frequently.

I think that may be why Savasana is hard for some
people. Letting go, if only for a few minutes, is hard.

Although I will tell my yogis to let go of
something that is eating at them, I also tell them to
know that it is hard, but they have to take care of

themselves. I will teach classes where we simply stop and breathe for a couple of minutes, sitting or standing. We will do this several times, too, maybe doing some specific breathing exercises. Sitting and breathing is a good way to begin a class, end a class, and prepare for Savasana.

We can let go without actually being told to let go.

43. LAUGH, OR CRY

I try to inject humor into my yoga classes. I want everyone to have fun and enjoy themselves. I also want them to know that it is okay to laugh; that sometimes yoga shouldn't be taken that seriously. The yoga room isn't a sacred or hallowed place. It is a room where we practice yoga.

Laughter is also a good way to learn. If I tell them to hold their hands like they are holding a bowl of Snickers, they laugh. I tell them it could be fruit, but I prefer Snickers. Likewise, if we are using the yoga straps in a Seated Forward Bend (Paschimottanasana) I remind them that they aren't trying to stop a stagecoach. Hold onto the strap, but not with a death grip. (Let go…)

Once, before I was an actual yoga teacher, we were working on a Wide-Legged Forward Bend (Prasarita Padottanasana). We were getting pretty deep and heads were getting close to the floor. The teacher had us hold the pose and then she told us to start bringing our feet closer together, lengthening the distance from our heads to the floor. She had us bending over and our legs were getting it. All of a sudden, a woman in class blurted out, "Oh sh*t!" Of course we laughed. We were thinking it anyway; she just said it.

On the other spectrum, yoga might be a time to let go and cry. I've never had anyone break down and sob in my class, but I know there have been tears. Once when we were working with the balls on myofascial release, a woman came up to me after class. She had been suffering with tightness and had not been able to find a relief. Until she used the balls. She said while we were laying on our backs with the balls between our shoulder blades, she felt instant relief and tears started flowing.

I have had my moments, too. The first time was in 2015 when Susan, my horse trainer friend, died suddenly from a heart attack. I played an M83 playlist, a suggestion from a friend in class. However, it was all I could do to get through that class. "Wait" is a beautiful M83 song. I had to skip it for that day and my friend asked me after class why I didn't play it. I burst into tears and told her about Susan. I told her I just couldn't play that song yet. She understood.

Another time, two times actually, were in 2019. I had rescued Casey, a Treeing Walker Coonhound in 2017. In the summer of 2019 he was diagnosed with cancer. He got worse and worse. I had just had my hip replaced and was back to teaching when he got worse. My dog-lover friends in class were concerned. Right before class was about to begin, a friend asked me how he was doing. I shook my head and my eyes immediately filled with tears.

"Sorry," she said.

I nodded my head and then managed to somehow tell everyone to lay on their backs and start their yoga breath for a few minutes. When they did, I did, too, and tears slid down my cheeks like a small river. I had to keep it together to teach, and somehow I did.

The same thing happened the next week during my evening class. It was a smaller class and three of my dog-lover friends were there, so I had a good cry with them after I managed to teach a class. Casey went to heaven the next day and I got subs for all of my classes and cried all day.

We laugh and cry for a reason. It is a release.
Yoga is a release. They go together.

44. WATCHASANA

There are times in yoga class that someone should
just stop and watch what I am doing. I like to call this
"Watchasana."

I might offer Watchasana if I need to show the
class something before they attempt it, such as Crow
Pose. Crow Pose is also a good pose to simply
practice Watchasana. Visual learners might need to
see it first. Yogis who might be a little timid or
hesitant about Crow Pose are good candidates for
Watchasana.

Along with modifying a pose or doing a different
pose, I will offer the choice of Watchasana. Yogis
can simply opt out or avoid a pose for whatever
reason and watch. I don't mind a bit.

I've practiced Watchasana in several workshops.
I'm a visual learner and I also appreciate watching
others do poses I cannot do fully or at all. At one
particular workshop, we were working on Peacock
Pose (Mayurasana). Peacock is a hand balance.
Your hands are on the ground, turned toward your

knees. The elbows are bent backwards and the rest of
the body is lifted behind you, like a Plank. But the
hands are the only thing on the floor! Except in my
case. My butt was on the floor because I was
perfecting Watchasana, admiring the teacher in his
perfect Peacock Pose, but knowing this pose isn't for
me. I tried. I simply can't do it.

You've heard the expression, "Hide and watch!"
Well, in yoga, you don't have to hide. You can
simply watch.

45. LIVE YOGA OFF THE MAT

As I have mentioned, everyone is included in my
classes. The focus is on breathing, healing, feeling
better, being better, laughing, de-stressing, and letting
go. I want everyone to remember to take that with
them when they leave the class. Use your breath as
you go about your day. Do some portable poses.

More importantly, try to maintain a positive and
happy attitude. Have an attitude of gratitude. There
is always something to be thankful for and if you take
the time to be thankful, you will find at least one
thing and many more, I'm sure. While you're
counting some blessings, think of some things that

make you happy. Happiness is a choice and I choose it. I can't understand people who can never see the good in things; all they do is gripe. When they enter a room, even a yoga room, you can feel the life and joy being sucked right out of you. How miserable it must be to be so negative and grumpy all of the time.

Take an inventory and get rid of stress. Oh, it's easy to get stressed out about things. While I don't believe we can ever be completely stress-free, perhaps we can be "stress lite." Avoiding certain encounters, events, and even people can help reduce our stress level. This can increase your happiness level, as well.

Just as you modify poses, modify your attitude and circumstances. Perhaps the line at the store is too long. Can you control it? No. You can breathe, though. You can also be kind to the clerk, who is probably overwhelmed. It's easy to lash out. It's also easy to smile. Pay a complete stranger a compliment. Let someone ahead of you in traffic. Wave your whole hand at them, not just your middle finger, if they fail to acknowledge your generosity.

Church isn't only on Sunday mornings. We are Christians 24/7 and we should act like it. The same goes with yoga. While I don't share the beliefs, especially political ones, with many people in my classes, I'm still nice to them. I also have a strict rule that there will be ZERO political discussions during yoga.

At the end of the day, when you are about to go to sleep, would you rather remember a hostile reaction you had to someone, especially when it was beyond their control, or would you rather remember that you reacted kindly to them? Which one will help you sleep better? Oh I know that some people are just begging for a butt-chewing. Believe me! I know it! Take a few breaths. Think of something happy. Say a quick prayer. You probably won't score 100% all of the time. Be kind anyway.

46. NAMASTE Y'ALL

Namaste (nom-uh-stay) is a greeting and farewell, like Aloha. At the end of class when we are seated and taking our last moments of deep breath, silence, and peace, I offer the class a chance to be thankful, count a few blessings, think of something that makes them happy, or to say a prayer. I have them bring their hands to their hearts in prayer. Then I will thank everyone for practicing yoga with me, bow to them, and say, "Namaste."

If a holiday is coming up, I'll add a Happy or Merry Whatever. If there is a big football game, I'll say "Go Pokes" much to the chagrin of my Sooner yogis. Everyone agrees, though, when I say, "Go Thunder" or "Thunder Up!"

I was told that Namaste means "I see the light in you and you see the light in me." A woman from India in one of my classes told me it means, "I see God in you and you see God in me." I like that. That is what I tell people now when they ask me what Namaste means.

Namaste!

47. FIND YOUR PLACE

Yoga can be like church in a couple of ways. The first way is that, despite being inclusive and accommodating, your physical place for your mat can be as territorial as the pew you sit in at church. That is just a fact, and it happens in every yoga class that I teach.

Most people are accommodating and "flexible" in that a newcomer who unwittingly gets someone's sacred spot is spared the public humiliation and branding of a scarlet letter. They will even happily find a place on the other side of the room, gasp, and continue their practice without batting an eye. Most people.

I have seen people actually move someone else's mat because they dared to put it in the spot that is religiously taken by the "yoga mat mover." There are no apologies, but rather they say, "This is MY spot!" I have witnessed this in church, too. It is embarrassing, shameful, and un-Christian.

To keep a little humor going, if someone is late and they are looking for a spot, there are always spots up front by me. I extend an invitation to them and tell them it is just like church; there is always room on the front row!

Aside from the physical location of your mat, people will find a yoga class and teacher(s) where they feel comfortable, enjoy, and fit in. Their needs are being met. Kind of like church. There are some people in my class who come to as many classes of mine that they can, at different YMCAs. I truly appreciate that. One of them told me that she was my "groupie." We had a great laugh but again, it reaffirms that I am teaching what people like and need and can do.

When people ask me about other teachers, I tell them to try their class. I will not disparage or gossip about another teacher. When I am asked about a different style of yoga, I tell them to try it. When they ask me if I've ever taken a Bikram class (the room temperature is 105 degrees and 26 poses are practiced twice), I tell them yes. I actually took the class just so I could tell my yogis about it. I also tell them the truth about the class: I did not like it but it is great for stretching, there is the danger of overstretching and tearing a muscle, I sweated so much I looked like I had crawled out of a river; and, my cardiologist said for me not to attend hot yoga classes. I don't discourage them because there are people who absolutely love Bikram classes. You won't know until you try.

48. MUSIC FOR THE SOUL

Music is a big part of yoga for me. Most of the time, I play "yoga" music. I will also play classic rock. To me, it is great for yoga. However, not everyone likes it. Soft rock, like Dan Fogelberg and James Taylor, is also pleasant for yoga as well.

Once I played the soundtrack to *The Big Chill* at one particular class. Boy did I catch it! "Thank God that is over!" "I thought this class would never end!"

"I hope she never plays that music again." Okay.
Got it! For this class, I stick to the standard yoga
music. No classic rock. No soft rock.

Other classes love different types of music.
They've even given me suggestions. I've told them
I'll play anything except rap or jazz because I do not
like rap or jazz.

I never want my classes to be boring. So around
holidays, I play the appropriate music for certain
classes. Most classes like my Halloween playlist, but
some yogis in one particular class (hint: I mentioned
them in paragraph 2) are very divided about it. One
woman came up to me and asked if I was going to
play that Halloween music in every class. I couldn't
resist and responded by telling her it wouldn't be
Halloween every day. She got a little huffy and I told
her that I would not play it again. Fortunately,
everyone seems to like Christmas music. Even the
class in Paragraph #2 seems to enjoy the quiet
Christmas music. Not "Run Run Rudolph" or
anything like that, though; I save that for my core
class. I also have a Motown playlist so we have
Motown Mondays, just not in the aforementioned
yoga-music-only-see-paragraph-2 class.

Along with certain music themes, I will focus on
themes such as Warrior Wednesday, incorporating the

various Warrior poses. I also teach Twisty Tuesday where we work on twists. Pigeon Pose has been the theme, especially for my Pigeon Coop ladies (see #49).

49. TEACHING WHAT MY YOGIS LIKE

Long ago, I learned to read the room before starting class. This was set in stone once when everyone was seated, getting ready for class to start. I had my class all planned out and told everyone to stand up and start in a Forward Bend (Uttanasana), with bent knees. There was a loud, collective, disgruntled, groan from everyone.

"UGGGHHHH!"

"Okay!" I said. "You win. Stay seated."

My yogis were happy. And I changed up the class. I have never had everyone stand up and bend over again to start a class. Everyone likes to hear the story, too.

Many times before class begins, I ask everyone what they would like to work on. Or not work on. Shoulders and hips and low backs are usually the normal requests. I have also had people tell me that something in particular that we did really helped. So when I see that person in class, I incorporate that into the practice as well.

There is a group of women, the dog lovers, in one of my classes that absolutely love Pigeon Pose. I love Pigeon Pose, too. So when all or part of this group, affectionately known as the Pigeon Coop, is present, I make sure to throw in a Pigeon Pose. I get sighs of pleasure, "ahhhs," "yeas," and even applause at times. Sometimes I surprise them when I do it. I have made it the second pose of the practice, put it in the middle, or close to the end. Sometimes we do Pigeon Pose twice, much to their delight. However I learned if I wait too long, things can get a little testy. "It's about time!" or "Finally!" are usually the responses. I have even incorporated all manners of Pigeon Pose into class at times: Reclined Pigeon, "regular" Pigeon, Seated Pigeon, Cradle the Baby, and Pigeon at the Wall.

Warrior Poses were requested recently. So that's how I structured the class, going through all five Warriors (I, 2, 3, Humble, and Reverse) at various times and then in one big finale, going through all five in one long flow. My yogi was happy. She told me she loves Warriors and we seem to not do them enough. Noted. Even though I thought I taught them frequently, I will teach them even more frequently now, especially when she's in class. Gotta keep my yogis happy!

50. ALWAYS KEEP LEARNING

There isn't a person alive who knows everything there is to know about yoga, just like there isn't a person alive who knows everything about anything. Yoga evolves. Teaching yoga evolves.

I enjoy attending workshops, reading about yoga and watching "how to" videos or listening to podcasts about it. I want to keep learning so I can teach it to my classes and they can learn. Usually, when I've learned a new "trick" I'll tell my class that I just went to a workshop.   I'll hear groans and "Oh, great…" Even if I haven't learned a new "trick," just mentioning that I went to a workshop elicits the moans and groans. However, many of the things I learn and in turn, teach, are surprisingly well met once they realize they do not have to stand on their heads and juggle.

Much of what I learned in the beginning of my yoga career now has to be unlearned, or more simply, just taught a new way, because teachers are discovering that what was once taught as "gospel" actually leads to injuries. I'm not afraid to admit to my class that there is another way, a safer way, and that the "old" way is moot.

One example of this is starting a practice with a forward bend, which I mentioned in #49. The spine needs to be properly warmed up so actually, starting off with a forward bend is a no-no. So my yogis were right, regardless of the fact that they just didn't want to stand up. Once I learned this in my workshop, I stopped teaching classes starting with forward bends. In fact, once we do add a forward bend, I tell the class to really bend their knees, especially if this is their first forward bend of the day. I also remind them in their standing forward bends to look down as they bend over and to keep looking down until they stand up. That way the neck is not compromised. This is a nugget I gleaned from a workshop about the neck, and share with them repeatedly. It is also practical advice for picking something up off the floor and I remind them of that as well. Safety first!

Another former way of teaching was how to get on the sit bones in a seated pose. I learned, and it was taught, that to properly get the sit bones on the floor, you needed to pull your glutes (gluteus maximus…butt flesh) up. Actually, that pulls on the hamstrings, which connect to the sit bones and down to the backs of the knees. So to safely teach getting on the sit bones, roll your inner thighs towards the outside and pull them out. (Push your inner right thigh under the thigh and pull it out on the right side.) This gets you on the sit bones without harming the hamstrings. This might have been helpful in the aforementioned "personal space violation" workshop.

Whatever your passion or your job is, never stop learning. If you only learn one detail, even a small one, it is so worth it and can be extremely valuable. Learn it and pass your knowledge on to others.

Namaste.

OTHER RESOURCES:

Hatha Yoga Illustrated by Martin Kirk, Brooke Boon, and Daniel DiTuro

The Roll Model by Jill Miller
https://www.tuneupfitness.com

Yoga For Equestrians by Linda Benedik and Veronica Wirth

YogaUOnline Education https://yogauonline.com

READ OTHER

50 THINGS TO KNOW

BOOKS

50 Things to Know

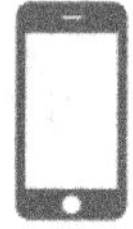

Stay up to date with new releases on Amazon:

https://amzn.to/2VPNGr7

50 Things to Know

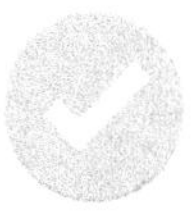

We'd love to hear what you think about our content! Please leave your honest review of this book on Amazon and Goodreads. We appreciate your positive and constructive feedback. Thank you.